MOVE, PLAY, GROW!

Move, Play, Grow!

A Fun & Practical Guide to Support Your Baby's Milestones Ages Newborn to 2 Years

Dr. Kim Baugh, PT, DPT

ISBN: 979-8-218-81865-4

Library of Congress Control Number: 2025921480

Because of the dynamic nature of the internet, any web addresses or links contained in this book may have changed since publication and may no longer be valid. The views expressed in this work are solely those of the author and do not necessarily reflect the views of the publisher, and the publisher disclaims any responsibility for them.

Cover Design & Illustrations: Justin Hardin of Damascus Media
Editor: Dr. Joel Boyce of JCB Educational Services
Photo: VI Photography

Visit www.moveplayandgrow.com

For more resources to help you support your baby in reaching those important firsts.

☉This paper meets the requirements of ANSI/NISO Z39.48-1992 (Permanence of Paper)

1 2 0 9 2 5

*This book is dedicated to my two beautiful daughters—
my "why's" in life. The two of you inspire and
motivate me to do the hard things.*

*To my husband, your encouragement, love, and belief
in me helped make this book possible. Thank you for
helping me turn this dream into a reality.*

*To my parents, thank you for a strong foundation and
a lifetime of unwavering support.*

*To all of the incredible children whom I've had the
privilege to work with, you all are the inspiration
behind this book.*

CONTENTS

This book is a resource guide for educational and informational purposes only. The information provided is based on a norm-referenced assessment tool, as well as knowledge gained through my professional experience over the years, which includes direct treatment and consultation and caregiver education. This book is not a substitute for a medical diagnosis. Please consult with a qualified and licensed healthcare professional in your area for any health concerns or before making any decisions related to the health or treatment of your child.

INTRODUCTION

"There are places in the heart that you don't even know exist until you love a child."

— Anne Lamott

Thank you for picking up your copy of *Move, Play, Grow! A Fun & Practical Guide to Support Your Baby's Milestones Ages Newborn to 2 Years*. Welcome to the fascinating, ever-changing, wonderful world of caring for a child. Your baby's first few years are full of learning and growth at a rate that will seem to be impossible to keep up with. While it may feel overwhelming at times, the good news is that each interaction, cuddle, and snuggle makes a big impact on your baby's ability to grow and thrive. In the first few weeks, months, and years, through positioning and movement, your baby's brain will make count-less connections at a rate higher than any other time in a person's life. With each new motor skill your baby learns, a new level is unlocked in their growth and development. Whether you are a new parent, educator, caregiver, or clinician, this book will help you unpack the why, when, and WINS of infant gross motor development.

Have you ever wondered why babies move the way they do? Have you ever worried about or questioned if your baby is reaching their milestones on time? Have you ever asked, "Is that normal?" Well, you're not alone. As first time parents, it's natural to have questions. It can be hard to know what is considered "typical" and what you should be concerned about. This book will not only help you learn what to expect, but it will also teach you when to expect certain milestones. It will also highlight common red flags to look out for to help you recognize early signs that your baby may benefit from extra support.

Are you tired of feeling dismissed or being made to feel that your questions are not valid? Do you stress about how to interact with your baby? Are you tired of playing the "wait and see" or "they will grow out of it" game?

As a pediatric physical therapist with over 20 years of experience, I've spent years helping little ones build strength, improve coordination and balance, and build confidence through movement. I have worked with hundreds of babies, children, and their families in a variety of pediatric settings. As a movement expert, specializing in infant and child development, one of the most important takeaways I want to share with you is that every baby moves at their own pace and in their own way. The range for what is considered typical is wide! I've also learned that family and caregiver support, along with effective positioning and movement strategies, are the biggest factors in a child's overall growth and development.

At the start of my career, as a new pediatric physical therapist, I can vividly remember that my course of action was planning my treatment plans well in advance. I would set up elaborate obstacle courses, and map out the exercises in the exact sequence in which I expected the child to do them. My goal was to get in a solid 45-50 minutes of hands-on therapy, but I realized after some experience and practice that my goals were not always what was needed. I had to learn to let the child steer their treatment sessions, based on what they needed for that day. I was learning that it was important to factor in the baby's and the family's activities the day prior to their therapy appointment in addition to the baby's current mood or demeanor. Was it nap time? Was the baby hungry? Was mom or dad overwhelmed? I started to discover that creating a safe space for parents to vent, ask questions, laugh, and learn more about their baby's development was just as (if not more) beneficial as checking off boxes of exercises completed for the day.

Instead of providing difficult-to-manage home exercise programs with multiple repetitions, I began to take time to show them simple practices and strategies that could be implemented into every day tasks (i.e. diaper changes). Decreasing stress centered around adding just one more thing to do and making it functional, works! With more experience, I began to build in more time for caregiver education, realizing that while my treatment sessions were very important, the carryover at home was the clutch piece in helping children reach their gross motor milestones.

I started to see how everyday practices, intentional movement, and exploration are really how a baby thrives and learns. Goodbye to copying and pasting my exercises! Say hello to baby and family-centered education and recommendations that fit the individual needs of the babies and families. Partnering with families and embracing the whole child, honoring their routines, cultural identity, and family dynamics is key to helping each child thrive.

I understand how overwhelming it can be, dealing with waitlists, struggling to find the right support for your baby's development, and experiencing the challenge of not having enough time with your healthcare provider to answer your questions. I have experienced moments when I was not fully able to answer parents' questions or walk through strategies and techniques as thoroughly as I would have liked. There were many times I wanted to provide support and answer questions outside of scheduled clinic hours, but I was often limited by time constraints and insurance restrictions. These experiences reinforced my drive to create meaningful, accessible resources for families beyond traditional settings.

When I shifted from working from protocols to meeting children and their families where they were, I learned that oftentimes, there can be improved outcomes in a shorter time frame. There can be improved carryover through working with the child in their natural environment (example: at home, daycare, or playground). I began to notice that consistent, short periods of meaningful movement in a functional way led to big results. I've come to understand that empowering parents and building their confidence are two of the most effective ways to support a baby's development. If the parent feels capable and supported, the chances are great that their baby will feel capable and supported, and they will be more likely to move, play, and grow!

Some common questions that I've heard consistently over the years are: "Is it normal or abnormal for my baby to do this? "Are they on track?" "Should I be worried?" Helping you by answering some of these questions is the true purpose of this book.

Throughout this book, each chapter will highlight some of the milestones you can expect during specific time frames. It is important to remember that every child is different, and they will develop in their own way and on their own timeline. This is a guide, not a rule book. Do not worry if your baby isn't doing all of the things mentioned in the particular chapter. It is common for babies to demonstrate scattered skills over the course of several months. Scattered skills may look like your baby hitting several milestones in one age group, while they are also practicing one or two skills in another age group. Give yourself and your baby time, space, and grace to grow.

I wrote this book to provide you a simple, fun, and practical guide to your baby's gross motor development from birth to two years old. This book is designed to help parents, caregivers, and educators understand the stages of gross motor development in infants and toddlers.

Inside, you'll find:

- What milestones to expect and when they should occur
- Easy, stress-free, and play-based activities to support your baby's movement
- Tips to encourage safe exploration
- Answers to common questions like, "Is this normal?" or "Should I be worried?"

This book is not about rushing milestones. It's about supporting your little one as they grow and explore through movement. There are ways you can help them along the way with lots of love, play, and a little bit of knowledge.

Consider this book as your "phone a physical therapist friend" lifeline for gross motor development. You will have questions on this parenting journey, but you will also be equipped to find the answers you need to support your baby.

My hope is that this book will help decrease your stress surrounding your baby's motor development in the first 2 years. The ways you and your baby play and move together now will have a lasting impact on how your baby grows. I want you to feel empowered, knowing that you are able to create space and allow grace for your baby to grow and thrive.

Happy playing!

~Dr. Kim~

CHAPTER 1

THE WHAT & WHY OF GROSS MOTOR DEVELOPMENT

"Play is the work of the child."
—by Maria Montessori

Let's start by explaining gross motor development. What is gross motor development? "Gross" means large or big, and "motor" means movement. These are the big muscle groups in your arms, legs, and core responsible for balancing and controlling your body position. Gross motor development is the ability to use large muscle groups to sit, crawl, climb, stand, walk, run, and jump. Having a strong gross motor skill set also helps support the body for improved speech output and fine motor tasks, such as feeding, writing, and tying your shoes.

Whether this is your first time around babies, or you're looking to refresh your knowledge, I invite you to explore with me the fascinating journey of how babies learn through motor development. Movement is more than just reaching physical milestones. It is an essential part of a baby's overall health and development. Gross motor development does not occur in isolation. It is deeply connected to all other areas of development, and it is an important piece to the development of the whole child.

It's okay if your baby isn't doing everything in the exact months as their chronological age. You may likely see a few skills across age groups. There may also be times in your baby's development that you may feel like they are not doing as much physically, but other areas are taking off. For example, your baby may appear to be stuck in sitting (not moving much in the sitting position) but you also notice that they are babbling and vocalizing more. That's still gross motor development at work. The core is stronger and allows better balance in sitting, which gives them a stable base to work on oral motor skills.

The goal is to see continued growth and a progression of skills. Imagine a high rise building. The foundation was set long before the upper floors were built. The same works for babies' gross motor development. There are foundational gross motor skills that a baby learns before moving on to the higher level skills. The length of time it takes for a baby to perfect those foundational skills before moving on varies, and oftentimes, it takes a while for them to perfect a skill. When a baby is learning a new skill, whether it is learning to hold their head up or taking their first step, repetition is key. Practicing a skill helps transition that movement from something that takes a lot of effort and thought to becoming automatic and smooth. Skills do not emerge overnight. They improve with daily opportunities and practice.

Gross motor development in babies follows a predictable pattern known as cephalocaudal development. The root words, "cephalo" means head, and "caudal" means tail, or lower part. A baby's development will follow a "head to toe" pattern.

This means that babies develop control over their bodies, starting with head control first, and gradually, they gain control, moving downward toward their feet. So keep in mind that your baby will first learn body control, starting with the head and moving to the shoulders, trunk, and then the legs. Remembering this top-down pattern of gross motor development is an important key in understanding how your baby will learn to move and control their body.

These chapters are based on a baby's chronological age. If your baby was born premature before 37 weeks gestation, adjust for your baby's prematurity. This is called an adjusted age. You should expect your baby's gross motor development to track according to their adjusted age, *not* their chronological age. Typically, when tracking a baby's progress toward their gross motor development, a premature, preterm baby's age is adjusted up to age four.

An example calculating adjusted age:

Today's date: 5/11/25

Baby's birth date: 1/11/25

Baby's original due date: 3/11/25

Chronological age = 4 months old (based off of birthday)

Adjusted age (based on prematurity & original due date) = 2 months old

---

Using the example above, a baby's progress should be tracked according to a two-month-old, not a four-month-old. If your baby is developing ahead of schedule, that's great. If not, it is still okay. In line with evidence-based practices, tracking a baby's milestones according to their adjusted age is the gold standard of measuring how well a premature baby is developing for their first few years of life.

One of the best things you can do to help your baby reach those important, early motor milestones is to limit the use of containers (i.e. swings, bouncers) outside of the time needed to safely transport them from one place to the next. Giving your baby lots of floor time (especially in the earlier months) will provide opportunities for them to stretch and strengthen those muscles they will need later for bigger skills such as sitting and crawling.

CHAPTER 2

TUMMY TIME

"Children are a gift from the Lord. They are
a reward with Him."
—Psalm 127:3 (New Living Translation)

How many times have you been told to make sure you get in tummy time with your baby? How many times have you heard your pediatrician say that tummy time is important? How many times have they asked you, "Are you doing tummy time?" I am sure you have felt like answering their question with a question. Oftentimes, the recommendation for tummy time is thrown at you without further explanation. You may be thinking, *Ok, sure. " We can give it a try, but when can we start trying tummy time?" How much tummy time does my baby need?* You may have tried to follow the "tummy time rule," but your baby hates it. They cry or wriggle and arch their bodies, attempting to end what seems to be a very unpleasant and uncomfortable experience for them. This leads you to then ask, "Why are we even doing this?" What is so special about tummy time?"

Tummy time is a very important activity for newborn babies because it helps build the strength and coordination that they need to grow and develop. Your baby's muscles are working hard during tummy time, specifically strengthening their neck, shoulder, arms, and back muscles. These muscles are key players for skills such as controlling their head in unsupported positions, rolling over, pushing up through their arms, sitting, and crawling.

Tummy time also works on visual motor skills, giving your baby a different field of vision to strengthen their eye muscles. It encourages your baby to take in their environment from a different vantage point.

Whenever your baby spends time on their tummy, it relieves pressure from the back of their head and body. This is particularly helpful in preventing flat spots from forming on the back of the baby's head, which can happen if they spend too much time lying on their backs. The flattening of a baby's head, which is called plagiocephaly or "flat head syndrome," is a medical condition that can cause difficulties outside of their general appearance. Plagiocephaly can lead to other issues such as asymmetry of facial features (most commonly the eyes and ears), tightness of the neck and shoulder muscles on one side of the body, and impaired visual tracking as a result of tight neck muscles.

Tummy time can start on day one of your baby's birth. When your baby is placed on your chest after delivery for the first time for skin-to-skin contact, that's tummy time. The benefits of skin-to-skin contact go beyond just being good practice for tummy time. Other advantages include strengthening the bond between you and your baby, reducing stress and pain for both you and your baby, and helping to regulate your baby's body temperature.

Now that you've conquered your first tummy time session, keep practicing once you and your baby are home. Your newborn baby may not be ready to lie completely flat on the floor just yet, and that's okay. Build tolerance by holding your baby chest-to-chest while you're sitting upright or comfortably reclined. Be sure to support your baby's head and neck at all times in these positions. Early tummy time can also be done with your baby lying on their belly across your lap. Keep your baby's nose clear by making sure they are lying on their belly with their head turned (cheek down, not forehead down) and looking toward either side. Alternate which side you turn your baby's head each time to keep both sides of those head and neck muscles stretched out equally.

Having consistency with tummy time is one of the easiest things you can do to help your baby learn and develop skills needed later for those bigger gross motor movements, while also preventing plagiocephaly. A few minutes of tummy time each day in short intervals will make a big difference. As your baby gets stronger and more comfortable, you can slowly increase the amount of time they spend on their belly.

Knowing when to practice tummy time is important for your baby's success and safety. Tummy time should always be supervised and done while your baby is awake and alert. Certain times of the day may be more challenging for tummy time, such as when you have recently finished feeding them or when your baby is feeling gassy.

If your baby has reflux or experiences feeding

challenges, they may initially find tummy time uncomfortable. There are gentle ways to help them build tolerance over time. Allowing them at least 30 minutes after a feeding and keeping your baby slightly elevated during tummy time may help make the experience more comfortable. This approach can also help reduce the chance of your baby spitting up after a feeding. If your baby appears distressed and difficult to console during tummy time by arching their neck and back excessively or crying throughout the entire time, take a break, B-R-E-A-T-H-E, and revisit tummy time later.

Helpful tips for tummy time success include:

- Practice tummy time during your baby's awake, alert state. Do not force tummy time or push through bouts of crying. Avoid practicing tummy time when your baby is hungry, tired, or distressed.

- Laying your baby on your chest while you're reclined on the couch or chair for a few minutes or while you're sitting comfortably in a chair for a few minutes counts! Lying flat on the floor is not the only way to practice tummy time.

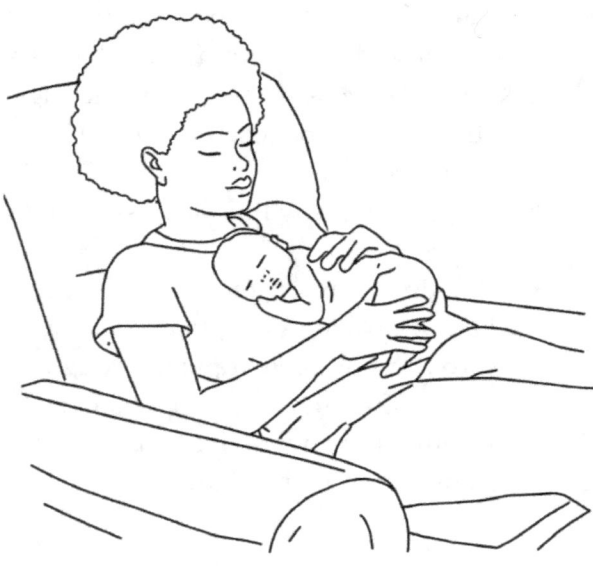

- Incorporate it into everyday position changes. For example, after changing your baby's diaper, gently roll them onto their belly and let them hang out there for a few seconds. When you incorporate this practice at each diaper change, those short intervals will add up throughout the day.

• Avoid tummy time right after a feeding. Allow time (at least 30 minutes) for your baby's stomach to settle. Oftentimes, discomfort associated with reflux limits the baby's ability to lie on their belly.

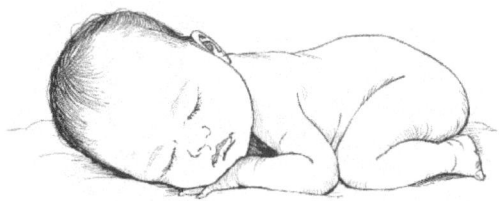

- Use a Boppy pillow or towel roll and place it under your baby's arms with their elbows tucked over the roll to help take pressure off their belly and assist them with lifting their head.

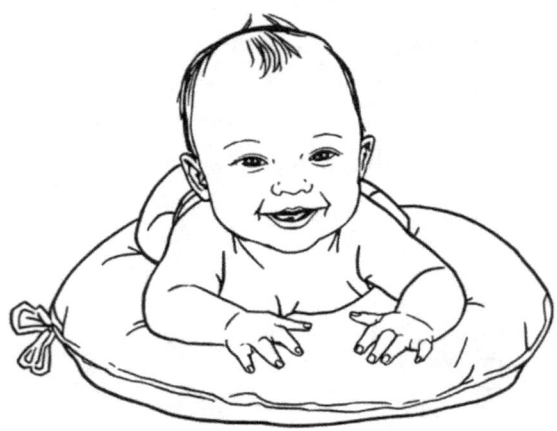

BUILDING BLOCK:

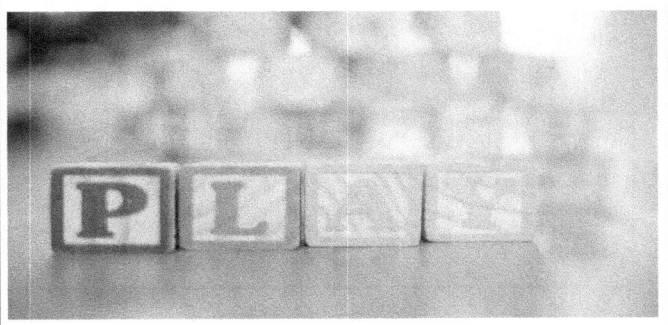

Let's move!

It's your baby's first diaper change of the morning. During the diaper change, roll them onto their belly for a minute or two as tolerated. Diaper on, check! It's time to get dressed. It's a onesie only kind of day, and after you pull your baby's onesie down over their head, gently roll them onto their belly to shimmy it down their back and straighten it out. Give your baby a few seconds to a minute to take in this new position. Then, gently roll them back onto their backs to finish the dressing process. Take a moment to sing, talk, and just bond with your baby during this process. Guess what? You've just completed 2 tummy time sessions in a matter of minutes! You've also helped your baby build strength on both sides of their body and adjust to position changes! Your baby will have multiple diaper changes each day. Even if you're only able to incorporate tummy time into one to three of them, that's at least three to five minutes of the daily tummy time in those first few weeks.

Keep moving!

Tummy time ways to play include:

- Snuggle with your baby and allow them to lie on your chest. Help them keep their hips and knees slightly flexed while securing them under their bottoms.
- Lie on the floor facing your baby. Talk to them, sing, laugh, and enjoy each other's company while encouraging your baby to lift their head to make eye contact with you. The lifting of the head will be brief and uncontrolled at first. Your baby may be able to lift their head suddenly, but they may not be able

to lower it with control. Make sure your baby is on a blanket or soft material to protect their head.

- Lie your baby on their belly and over your lap with their head and body resting comfortably on your leg. Alternate the direction of your baby's head with each lap tummy time session. This will ensure that your baby is looking both directions and working towards symmetry.

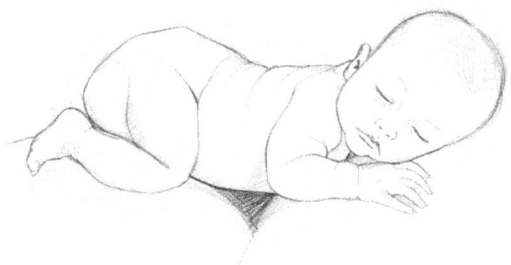

- Sometimes, lying your baby completely on the floor is extremely hard for newborn babies. Using the techniques provided will help your baby progress with tolerance to tummy time.

Chapter 3

Newborn to 3 Months

> *"Sometimes, the littlest things take up the most room in your heart."*
>
> —Winnie the Pooh

Your baby is home, and you may be thinking, *Now what? What things can a newborn baby do? What should I expect a baby to do outside of eating, sleeping, and pooping?* The answer is–a lot! Even during the early days, your baby's brain and body are working overtime to adjust to life outside of the womb. Every moment is a part of their growth, learning, and development. Don't underestimate the importance of touch and positioning. Your baby is learning how to control their body in space, and they are working on fine-tuning their sensory system. Our sensory system is made up of the senses we use to take in information from the world around us, like sight, sound, smell, taste, and touch. It also includes our vestibular system (which helps us with balance and movement) and our proprioceptive system (which helps us understand where our body is in space). The more sensory input your baby receives (i.e. movement experienced while being held in different positions and talking to your baby), the more motor output they develop, helping them grow stronger, more coordinated, and more aware of their body. Together, these systems help babies learn, move, and interact with their environment. Building relationships and establishing trust with you as their caregiver are the earliest ways of learning and wiring your baby's brain to tackle bigger tasks later in life.

During the newborn to three month stage, your baby is adjusting to the big, bright world they've been thrust into. The lights are bright. Surroundings can be loud, and there are no more cozy boundaries to keep their bodies snug as a bug. I like to call this the squirmy stage. Your baby will stretch and wriggle and begin turning their head to orient themselves to light, sounds, and smells.

While tummy time is important, being on their belly is not the only position a baby needs to grow and develop. Let's explore some of the ways your newborn baby can move, play, and grow.

Back: Your baby should be placed on their back to go to sleep at each nap time and at bedtime. Your baby's bed should be clear of all pillows, stuffies, toys, or blankets while they are sleeping. Being on their back is the safest way for your baby to sleep, and it reduces their chance of sudden infant death syndrome (SIDS).

Side lying: Your baby can be placed on their side in the first few days and weeks as well, with support behind their back, head, and neck. To make them comfortable and provide a boundary for better positioning and containment, you may place a towel roll underneath their bottom. Roll the towel into a loose "U shape" and place it underneath your baby's bottom, providing support on all sides of their body. Make sure you alternate sides and lay your baby on both sides for symmetry. This can be done in your lap with your baby's back against your belly or on top of a soft, padded blanket on the floor or bed, with supervision.

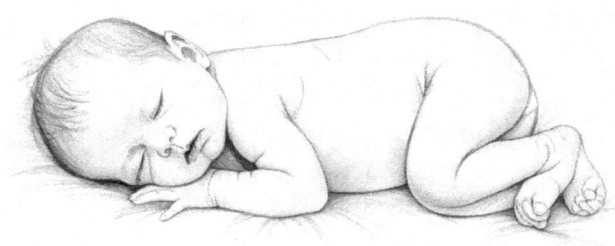

Belly: Remember tummy time? Yep, it's still a thing. Tummy time should happen often and daily. As your baby gets older and stronger, it will become second nature. Experiencing a variety of positions throughout the day will not only help your baby's muscles for strengthening and stretching, but it will also open up their world to new exploration through visual and auditory stimuli.

Newborn to 3 months milestones to expect include:

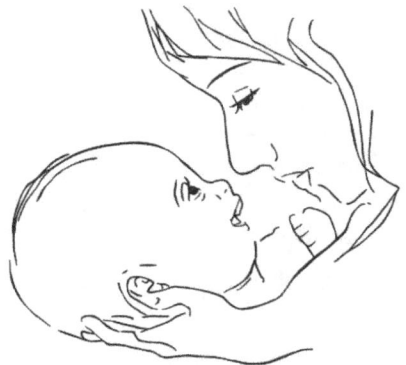

- Tracks *(tracking means to follow with your eyes)* an object in their line of sight. Move slowly and keep your face or toy that your baby is tracking within a few inches from their face.
- Brings their hands together.
- Brings their hands to their mouth.
- Turns their head toward voices and other sounds.
- While lying on their stomach, your baby will be able to raise their head briefly.
- While lying on their back, they may bat at or reach for objects.

- Can hold a small, lightweight object in one hand for a few seconds.
- Rolls from their side to their back.

Ways to play:

- Use tummy time to allow your baby time and space to work on establishing head control and lifting their head while you interact with them.
- Help your baby bring their hands together. Playing patty cakes or hand over hand, nursery rhyme songs. Perform gentle stretches to your baby's arms and legs. Slowly stretch your baby's arms and legs up and down and

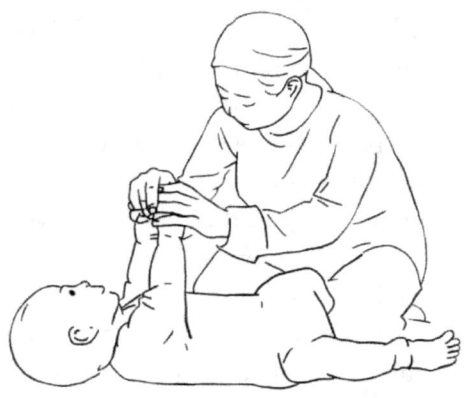

across their tummy (both sides). You can do this while getting them dressed or undressed each day.

- Give your baby time on both sides of their body each day. Lay down with them for face-to-face interactions or place a small baby-safe mirror a few inches in front of their face for them to watch themselves.
- Alternate sides while feeding (both breastfeeding or bottle fed) and change sides each time you feed your baby to work towards symmetry and visual tracking.
- Every day, practice handling your baby, including rocking, holding, and swaddling them. More input = more output. The more you touch, position, and talk to your baby, the more opportunities they have to work on body control, movement, and communication skills.

4 TO 6 MONTHS

"Play is the highest form of research."
—Albert Einstein,

If newborn to three-month-old babies are the "squirmers" and "wrigglers," by the time they reach the four to six month old age, they become "rollers" and "wobblers." With the introduction of rolling, your baby's world opens up to moving in space and venturing out beyond where they were placed. That first roll from their side to their back that may have looked like a mistake when momentum took over from a lift of their arm becomes intentional over time. Babies tend to roll from their bellies to their backs first as this takes less strength to accomplish. Rolling from their backs onto their belly requires more core and shoulder strength to reach up and over against gravity.

They are also beginning to show signs of being able to sit independently, initially wobbling and toppling over until they master the skill. Each wobble and loss of balance while learning to sit is practice toward independent sitting. While practicing sitting balance, keep your baby safe by placing pillows and other soft buffers near them to protect them when they lose their balance.

As your baby begins to spend less time laying on their backs and more time sitting upright, it is still important to keep an eye out for symmetry. Encourage your baby to turn their heads toward both directions when interacting with them. An easy way to work on strengthening both core muscles and working on neck rotation is to sit your baby on your lap facing the side. Give the support needed for safety and balance at their trunk while encouraging them to look both directions.

4 to 6 month milestones to expect include:

- Rolling over belly to back and back to belly.
- Kicking their legs and moving their arms with more control (not just a wiggle).
- Making swimming motions while on their belly.
- Transferring an object from one hand to the other.
- Banging two objects together in midline (midline is the middle of the body).
- Being able to sit with minimal support at their trunk.
- Sitting momentarily (a few seconds) while propped on their hands.
- Scooting and pivoting on their belly.
- Increasing interest in toys (functions, sounds, and textures).
- Lifting their head when lying on their back. Babies will tuck their chins and begin to lift their head when being pulled into a sitting position from laying flat.

Ways to play in the four to six month age range include:

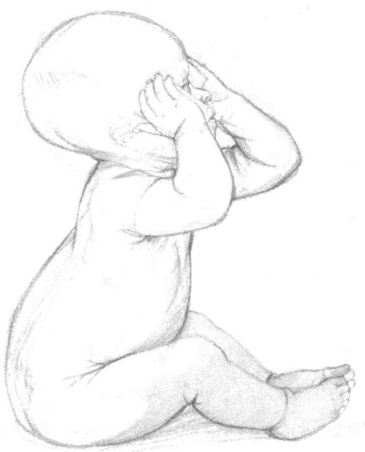

- Work on independent sitting using a Bobby pillow to help prop them up. This will help with strengthening the arms and core when the baby pushes into the Boppy pillow while also providing a soft, safe place to land.
- Place your baby in a laundry basket or large box to work on sitting balance. Save those diaper boxes. Drape a blanket over it and sit your baby inside with a toy. The box or basket will provide boundaries for

your baby to practice sitting and work through reaching and playing while learning to sit.

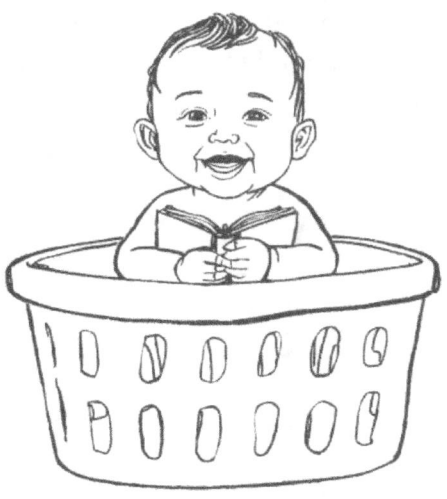

- Encourage rolling for transitions during dressing and diaper changes. Make it fun. Count 1-2-3 to signal that a change in position is coming.

- Play games including peekaboo, patty cake, and hand clapping games. This not only helps develop their use of both hands to play and learn, but it also encourages communication between you and your baby.

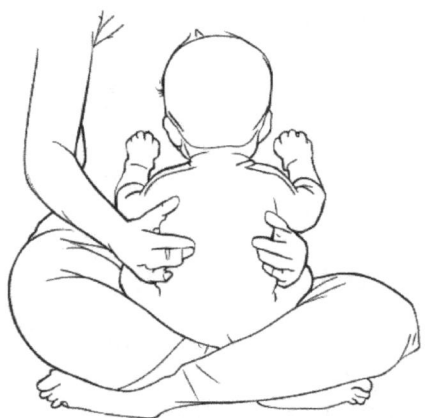

- Talking, laughing, and playing with your baby during this stage is great for visual tracking and alerting sights to sounds.

- Placing a lightweight toy just slightly out of their reach while they are on their belly will encourage reaching and eventually inching and crawling forward.

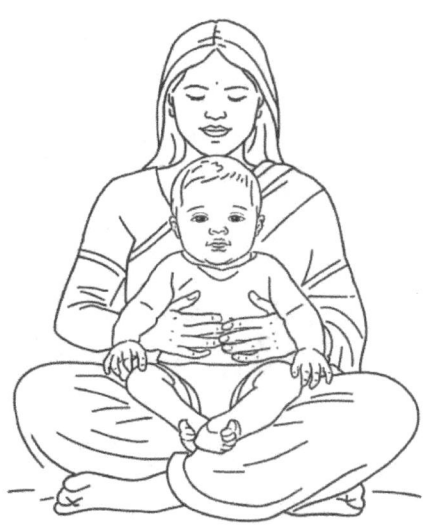

CHAPTER 5

6 TO 9 MONTHS

"Play gives children a chance to practice what they are learning."

—Fred Rogers

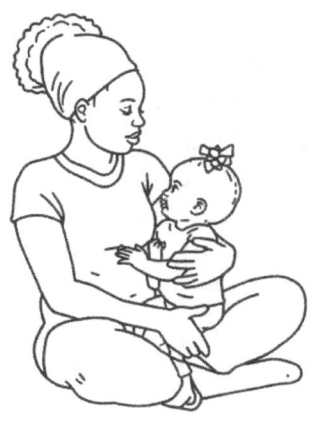

This age group is full of surprises and variation. Some babies may still be rolling as their main way of getting around, while others may be crawling, starting to pull themselves up to a standing position, or even taking their first steps.

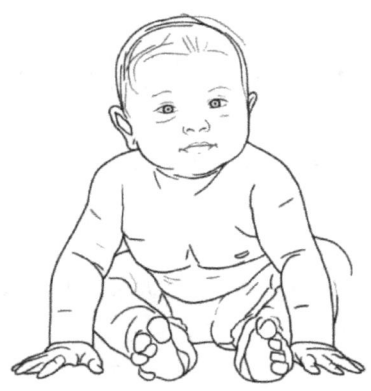

Some babies may appear to be stuck in a sitting position. They can sit for long periods of time, but they are not as confident moving into or out of a sitting position on their own. Some babies are content to sit and play in one spot, showing little interest to move beyond their base of support. While developing sitting balance is an important milestone, the ultimate goal is for your baby to progress to higher level activities, like reaching forward for a toy and returning back to an upright position without losing their balance.

BUILDING BLOCK:

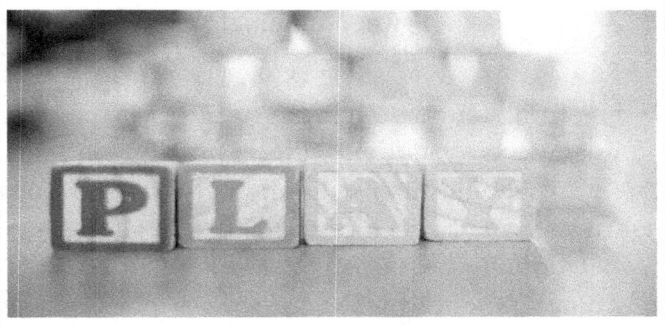

Let's Play!

If your baby seems to be "stuck" in the sitting phase, and they are able to sit for long periods of time, but they are not able to move into and out of the sitting phase, it may be time to introduce side sitting. Some babies will move in and out of the side sitting stage on their own, while others need a little help getting there. Side sitting is a great position for helping your baby build core strength. It also stretches tight hip muscles and encourages movement across the body, which is key for bigger skills like crawling and walking. Side sitting also strengthens the muscles needed for

improved posture–the ability to sit up tall and not rely on a rounded back to hold themselves up.
Keep playing!

A strong foundation in sitting also sets the stage for using their hands and fingers functionally, such as grasping and manipulating toys. As your baby grows stronger and more balanced in sitting, you can gradually begin to provide less support and encourage them to reach for toys or objects. This helps them build independence and control.

Since this is a big transition age group with the ability to move in and out of sitting, crawling, and some early walking, this is where you may see the biggest variation in what your baby is doing compared to other babies their same age. Scattered skills are common in this age group. Your baby may be doing a few things typically seen in the 6-9 month range, while still practicing skills from the 4-6 month stage. They may even surprise you with a skill from the 10-12 month range. Baby development does not always follow a straight path, and it's okay for babies to show a mix of abilities as they grow.

6 to 9 month milestones to expect include:

- Grabbing both feet and holding them when lying on their back.
- Bringing their feet to their mouth.
- Sitting for longer periods of time.
- Getting into a sitting position from lying on their back.
- Scooting, pivoting, or inching forward or in circles on their belly.
- Crawling.
- Pulling up to kneeling position.
- Moving into and out of sitting independently.
- Pushing up onto straight arms from their belly.
- Rocking back and forth on their hands and knees for a few seconds.
- Pivoting or scooting on their bottom.
- Bearing their weight through their arms and legs.
- Cruising along furniture or with both hands held.

This would be a good time to start baby proofing your home to keep your baby safe from electrical outlets, sharp edges/corners, and off of stairs.

Ways to play with your baby include:

- Giving your baby ample space to explore and crawl. Limit toys to fewer than three toys of interest to decrease distraction and overstimulation.
- Creating motor islands (ex: low lying safe ottomans connected to a couch or other safe furniture for your baby to practice pulling up to a standing position, cruising, and crawling within a safe area.

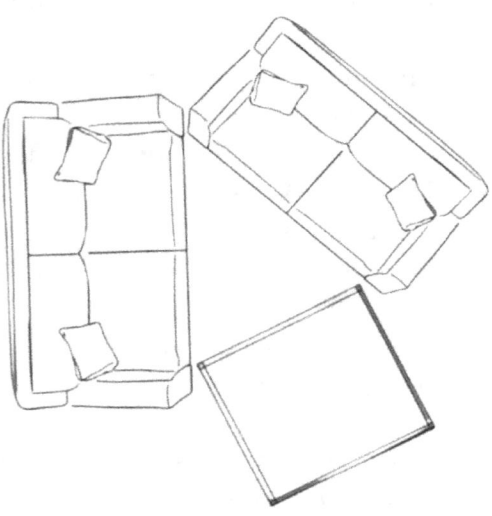

- Playing with a ball using a light-weight, baby-safe ball to roll back and forth to work on balance, visual tracking, and hand-eye coordination.
- Helping to stack large blocks. Showing your baby how to take toys/items out of containers (dumping, grasping and reaching).
- Placing your baby in a side sit position with a toy in front of them to encourage reaching on both sides.

CHAPTER 6

9 TO 12 MONTHS

"Almost all creativity involves purposeful play."

— Abraham Maslow

During this age, your baby may be in the early walkers group, or they may continue to work on their crawling technique. Is this a cause for concern? No. Both ways of mobilizing, mature crawling, and walking are considered within normal limits for 9 to 12 month olds. While some children will walk before the age of one, typical development is for independent walking to occur by the age of 18 months. Don't worry if your child is not walking by their first birthday; they still have time.

Babies in this age range may become experts in crawling. They soon realize that crawling is the fastest, most efficient way for them to cover ground. If your baby is crawling, but they are also showing signs of early walking (ex: pulling up to stand or being able to stand for a few seconds before falling), let them crawl. Try to avoid picking them up and placing them in a standing position. Let them work through the progression. They are showing signs that walking is on the horizon, and they are still well within the expected timeline.

There are so many benefits to crawling, and I am a huge advocate of encouraging this stage of development. Yes, there are babies who go straight into the walking stage and somewhat bypass the crawling stage. It's hard to force your baby back to the floor to crawl once their primary mode of mobility is walking, but I do want to cover some of the benefits of crawling.

Crawling is great for shoulder, arm, and core strengthening. Core strength is needed for so many things in life, including walking, standing, and balance. Crawling is also beneficial for hand-eye and overall coordination because it uses both sides of our bodies at the same time. Crawling also allows your baby to experience input through their hands and knees. The sensory input and subsequent output

44

helps with activities such as shoe tying, handwriting, and ascending/descending stairs with control.

Crawling is an amazing whole-body strengthening exercise from head to toe. Every single muscle group is needed for mature crawling. Attempting to skip this stage to get them to walk faster will not make your baby stronger or faster in the long run. It simply means that they skipped crawling, and they walked a little bit earlier than some of their peers. Early walkers do not always become early jumpers, faster runners or the first to learn to tie their shoes.

Crawling is an amazing milestone to help your baby to work toward bigger activities. If your baby is crawling, please allow them time and space to do so.

9 to 12 month milestones to expect include:

- Being able to sit for extended periods of time while playing with a toy.
- Transitioning from their belly to sitting and sitting to their belly.
- Bouncing while holding on to fingers, accepting weight through their legs, and pushing.
- Standing with support for longer periods of time.

- Standing independently for a few seconds.
- Cruising along furniture using one hand.
- Walking with one to two hands being held
- Walking while pushing a push toy.

Ways to play:

- Give the baby the floor. Now is the time for your baby to crawl, practice pulling up, go from kneeling to standing, or go from sitting to hands and knees or sitting to knees with support. An open area and a little floor space are all that are needed.
- Laundry baskets or large boxes can be used again. Place one end against the couch or wall to prevent tipping. Encourage your baby to climb in and out of it for a full body strengthening, coordination and motor planning activity. Pushing it across the floor, either on their knees or while standing to work on core strengthening and balance.

- Allow your baby to sit on a pillow placed on the floor to work on their trunk, strength, and balance. Place a couch cushion on the floor or on a large bed pillow. They should focus on sitting, crawling up onto and over, and standing on the pillow for strengthening and balance.

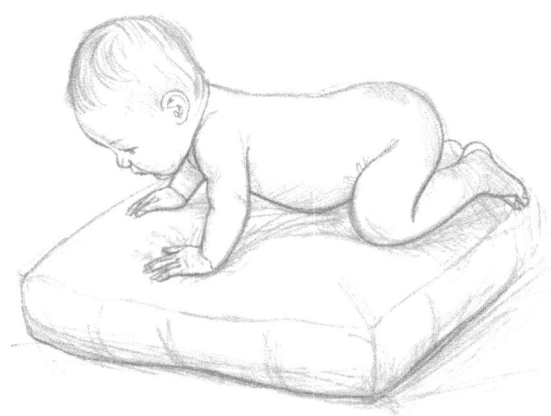

- Sit on the floor in front of your baby and place them in a standing position with their back against the couch or wall. Blow bubbles or have them reach for toys to keep them engaged. The prolonged standing and squatting to return to stand (as tolerated) is a great leg strengthening exercise.

Character 7

12 to 18 Months

"Every great journey starts with a single step."

—Maya Angelou

On your mark, get set, GO! Some of the early walkers have had lots of practice by now, and they are walking almost 100% of the time. Some babies may begin taking those first independent steps. The super crawlers are faster, and they can cover more ground.

Your baby will begin to explore beyond flat land and become more confident in climbing onto, over, and across obstacles. Try not to rush to pull your baby down from safe climbing or exploration.

49

When you allow trial and error to happen when your baby is trying to get to a desired location or grab a toy that isn't immediately within their reach, you are supporting the learning process. Motor planning and problem solving is taking place. Your baby will begin to self-correct and figure out what works and what doesn't work. Problem solving, motor planning, strengthening, and balance are all at work with each attempt to move their body.

> *"When a child is learning how to walk and falls down 50 times, they never think to themselves, 'Maybe this isn't for me."*
> —(Author Unknown)

12 to 18 months milestones to expect include:

- Being able to move from sitting to standing without support.
- Pushing up to stand from the floor without hands held or with surfaces.

- Walking with hands held (one or both).
- Standing for greater than 5 to 10 seconds independently.
- Creeping up stairs.
- Falling in a controlled way by slowly lowering themselves down vs. sudden (uncontrolled) landings.
- Squatting to pick up an object from the floor.
- Playing on their knees for longer periods of time.
- Holding a lightweight object while standing or walking.

Ways to play include:

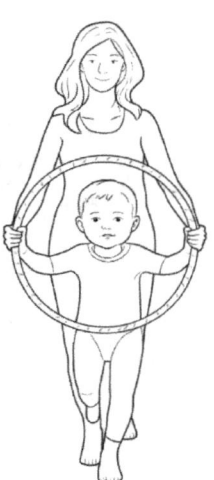

- Walking with your baby while providing handheld assistance. You can also use hula hoops, yoga rings, or pool noodles to help guide and support your baby while walking.
- Placing objects on a couch or slightly elevated surface to encourage standing.
- Using push toys for your baby to walk behind.

- Teaching safe stair mobility, creeping up stairs by crawling, and creeping backwards downstairs.

Here are some tips to keep your baby safe on the stairs:

1. Your baby should always CRAWL UP the stairs facing forward.
2. Teach your baby to CREEP backwards DOWN the stairs by first having them sit on the top stair.

Guide them onto their side and then onto their belly before creeping backwards down each step.

3. Remain with your baby each time they are on the stairs. Stay on a step or two below (behind) them in case of any falls.

4. Do not leave stairs open for free play or unsupervised use. Block both the top and bottom of the stairs with baby gates.

CHAPTER 8

18 TO 24 MONTHS

"Play is our brains favorite way of learning."
—Diane Ackerman

At this stage, your baby may go from creeping and crawling up stairs to walking up and down stairs. They are mature walkers, and early running may begin to emerge. Jumping and other higher level activities on their feet also emerge at this stage (i.e standing on one leg, hopping).

18 to 24 month milestones to expect include:

- Running forward 5-10 feet.
- Kicking a stationary ball.

- Throwing a ball while standing and maintaining their balance.
- Walking backwards.
- Walking heel to toe on the line.
- Walking upstairs with their hand on railing or handrail alternating feet
- Climbing on play equipment, couches, etc.
- When they are given paper and a crayon, they can spontaneously make marks on paper (ex: scribble).

Ways to play include:

- Encouraging active participation while getting dressed or taking clothing off. Talk through the steps and give directions. "It's time to lift your arm." "Use both hands."
- Participating in play groups. Babies this age will often participate in parallel play, meaning they may likely not play directly with each other, but within the same vicinity, side by side.

- Encouraging your baby to play in a squatting position.
- Picking up small objects or toys from the floor. Practicing squatting to stand from the floor for leg strengthening.
- Playing with toys that require "assembly" (i.e. large knob puzzles, twisting caps on and off, dumping things out and placing them back into a container).

CHAPTER 9

THINGS TO REMEMBER

"There is no such thing as a perfect parent.
So just be a real one."

—Sue Atkins

Now that you know what to expect, what happens if you're noticing a trend in a different direction? How will you even know if your baby is having difficulty with their motor skills? While all babies will develop at their own rate, there are red flags that may indicate your baby's need for intervention. There may be times when your baby does not demonstrate a skill within the expected age range. That is not always a concern, but given more time and practice to explore, you should expect to see that skill within the next age range.

For example, typically, a baby is able to sit, with varying degrees of balance and length of sitting time, between the ages of 4 to 6 months old. Your baby is 6 months old today, and they may not be able to sit for more than a few seconds before toppling over. While they did not meet the milestone of independent sitting in the 4 to 6 month range, they still have 3 months to work on it. If within the next 1-2 months, they meet that sitting goal at 8 months old, they are on the upper end of what is considered "typical". They are still within expected limits of that motor milestone.

If your child is having difficulty with a certain skill, or they are not demonstrating many of the skills leading up to a particular milestone, this may indicate a developmental delay. At that point, you should reach out to your healthcare provider.

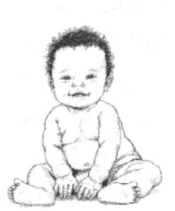 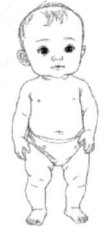 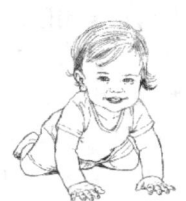

BUILDING BLOCK:

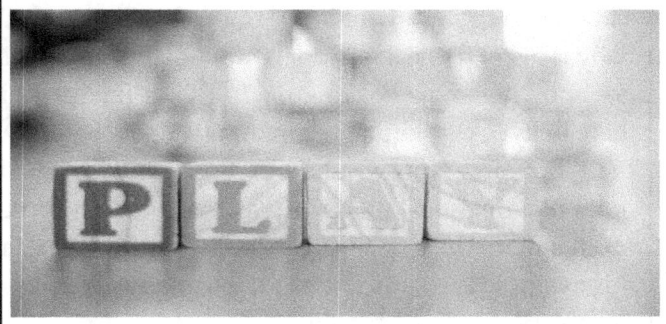

Let's Grow!

Let's consider this example. You and your 12-month-old baby attend a weekly playgroup at your local library. Several of the babies close to your baby's age (10-12 months old) are walking. Your baby is not.

Ask yourself the following questions. *Can my baby roll? Is my baby crawling?* If the answers are yes, your baby may not be walking at 12 months, but this is not considered developmental delay at this point. Your baby is mobile and they are building on the skills they need to walk (and likely sooner than you think).

Now, let's consider the following scenario. You

and your 12-month-old baby attend a weekly play-group at your local library. There are babies of the same age who are walking. Your baby is not. Your baby is also unable to sit independently. Your baby is not showing signs of crawling, moving forward on their belly, or scooting or pivoting while seated on their bottom. This would be considered a developmental delay. At this point, an intervention is recommended. The gap between sitting and walking in this example is significant enough to signal a need for extra support for your baby.

Below are key developmental milestones and associated red flags for each stage. Delays in achieving these milestones within the expected time frames may indicate the need for early intervention therapy services. Early support can make a big difference.

Newborn to 6 months:

- Having difficulty with rolling over front-to-back or back-to-front.
- Not bringing feet to hands or hands to mouth while lying on their back.

- Struggles to hold their head up, even when in a supported position.
- Difficulty sitting with or without support or excessive arching backwards or pushing out from a seated position.
- Unable to push their body off the ground with their arms while lying on their belly.

6 to 12 months:

- Not rolling.
- Showing no signs of crawling or movement while on their belly.
- Excessive arching or extension of the body. Increased time needed or difficulty bending arms or legs.
- Keeping one or both hands tightly fisted and clenched at all times.
- Shifting/moving weight or reaching only on one side of the body.
- Difficulty maintaining any position for greater than a few seconds.
- Unable to stand or bear weight through their legs with support.

1 to 2 years:

- Having difficulty or being unable to sit, crawl, or walk independently.
- Difficulty or unable to bring their hands together at their midline (the middle of their chest (body) without help.
- Unable to sit and/or maintain upright posture without support.
- Having difficulty bearing weight through both arms and legs.
- Showing a strong preference for using one side of the body.
- Cruising in only one direction; toward one side (i.e. only cruising to the right).
- Struggling with holding and releasing a lightweight object.
- Demonstrating excessive arching or extension in all positions.

Working closely with your pediatrician and your local pediatric physical therapist will be helpful in recognizing developmental delay. In some cases, children who are born prematurely or show signs of developmental delay will eventually "catch up" with their peers. With time, support, and early intervention when needed, many children close the developmental gap and thrive alongside their peer group. Even if your baby has received a medical diagnosis, they can and will still meet many of their motor milestones. Progress may happen at a different pace, and that's okay. With the right support and modifications, your child will continue to grow, develop, and achieve their individual goals. Early intervention is the best tool in helping your child achieve success in understanding and regulating their body's movement. This will help them not only in their gross motor skills, but it also will help with the overall development of the whole child.

CHAPTER 10

BUILDING BLOCKS, USING THE ABC'S

"While we try to teach our children all about life, our children teach us what life is all about."

— Angela Schwindt

The ABC method that I use can help you better understand whether your baby is developing within typical timeframes or showing signs of developmental delay. By meeting your baby where they are and at a pace that feels manageable for both of you, you can support their growth in a stress-free and confident way.

Try not to rush into correcting your baby's attempts at independent mobility or rushing them into positions that may be too difficult for them to maintain on their own. Taking a moment to do these 3 things can ease the fear and anxiety around your baby's development and help you find joy in the everyday moments. Each success counts, no matter how big or small.

A = Assess. Assess where your baby is developmentally. At which age range do they demonstrate the most gross motor skills? Do not rush ahead to the "next big thing".

B = Build. Build on the skills that they're currently working on. Progression over perfection.

C = Create. Create space for your baby to continue to grow and thrive. This may be physical space within your home. This could be a mental or emotional space. Free up mental space to invite others to help support your child's growth, such as their pediatrician, a pediatric physical or occupational therapist, or a pediatric speech therapist.

Use the ABC method, according to your baby's age, (adjust for prematurity if needed) and do a quick review of how your baby is doing using the following checklist:

Newborn to 3 months:

- Holds head in midline.
- Tracks an object right to left.
- Moves arms and legs (both sides).
- When lying on their back, they bat or attempt to reach toward a toy.
- Props up on elbows during tummy time.
- Is able to lift their head when lying on their belly.
- Brings hands to midline

4 to 6 months:

- Sits with support for extended periods of time.
- Sits independently for brief periods of time.
- Grasps feet with both hands.
- Brings feet to mouth.
- Brings hands to mouth.
- Begins to crawl.
- Rolls belly to back and back to belly.
- Holds and shakes a lightweight toy.

6 to 9 months:

- Is able to sit independently for extended periods of time.
- Can move in and out of a seated position.
- Moves forward in a circle or pushes backwards on their belly, either scooting or pivoting a few feet.
- Rocks back and forth on their hands and knees.
- Bears weight on hands while on their belly.
- Bears weight through their legs with hands held and/or supported.

9 to 12 months:

- Moves in and out of seated position.
- Cruises along furniture or with hands held.
- Stands independently for a few seconds.
- Walks a few feet when hands are supported.
- Lowers self from standing to a

seated position with control while hands are supported.

18 to 24 months:

- Walks independently.
- Stands for extended periods of time without falling.
- Walks while pushing a toy.
- Creeps up and down stairs.
- Is able to throw a ball while standing and maintaining balance.
- Walks up stairs with hands held.
- Walks in different directions, including backwards and sideways.
- Demonstrates emerging running skills.
- Kicks a stationary ball.

Your baby's brain is making millions of connections during their first three years of life. Play and emotional connections are two of the most powerful ways to support your baby's healthy development and growth. Allow yourself and your baby the space and grace to learn, grow, and thrive.

CONCLUSION

You are now more than ready to support your baby's development through intentional, purposeful play strategies. My hope is that you now have a better idea of when to expect milestones and what to look for if you need more support for your baby. During the first few years of life, our brains are the most active, and they develop faster than at any other time in our lives. Every loving interaction helps your baby's brain develop; early, positive experiences matter more than you think! Supporting your baby through play will not only improve their ability to reach their milestones through motor development, but it also teaches problem solving, body regulation, and social emotional growth. It also sets the stage of creating a safe space for them to learn and grow.

In this book, you learned strategies to help you support your baby's motor development. You learned:

- What developmental milestones to look for
- When to expect milestones
- What the red flags/signs of developmental delay are

Each day will bring something new for you and your baby to learn about each other. I now want you to progress forward and *move, play,* and *grow* with your baby. Don't let this book be the end of your journey. Take the things you've learned and continue to create an environment that promotes safe exploration and growth for that special little one in your life.

Happy playing!

Resources

The milestones and the age ranges in this book are based on the Peabody Developmental Motor Scales (PDMS-2), which is a standardized, norm-referenced assessment tool used to evaluate the fine and gross motor skills of young children from birth through age five.

Folio, M. R., & Fewell, R. R. (2000). Peabody developmental motor scales — Second edition (PDMS-2). Pro-Ed.

Here are some resources and organizations to contact if your baby needs extra support or you have further questions.

American Physical Therapy Association
3030 Potomac Ave., Suite 100
Alexandria, VA 22305-3085
800-999-2782

American Occupational Therapy Association
7501 Wisconsin Ave., Suite 510E
Bethesda, MD 20814-6519
301-652-6611

American Speech-Hearing-Language Association
2200 Research Blvd.
Rockville, MD 20850
800-638-8255

U.S. Center for Disease Control and Prevention
Early intervention programs
https://www.cdc.gov/act-early/early-
intervention/index.html
800-232-4636

March of Dimes National Office
1550 Crystal Dr, Suite 1300
Arlington, VA 22202

About the Author

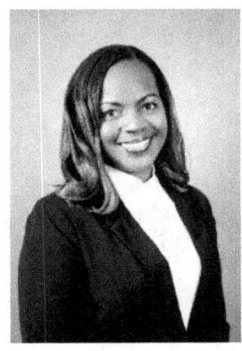

Kim Baugh is a neurodevelopmentally trained pediatric physical therapist with over 20 years of experience. She has worked in a variety of pediatric settings, including a NICU follow up clinic, children's hospitals and private clinics, promoting gross motor development, supporting families and improving the quality of children's lives. She has helped hundreds of little ones build their strength, improve their coordination and balance, and build confidence through movement. She is a school-based physical therapist, and is the owner and founder of Babies First, LLC, a pediatric physical therapy wellness and consulting company. She lives in Georgia with her husband and two teenage daughters.

Additional Information

Let's stay connected. Visit me on Instagram at @babiesfirstpt or visit www.moveplayandgrow.com to learn how to become a member of the Babies First community.